Addiction

The Bible

Allen Kelley

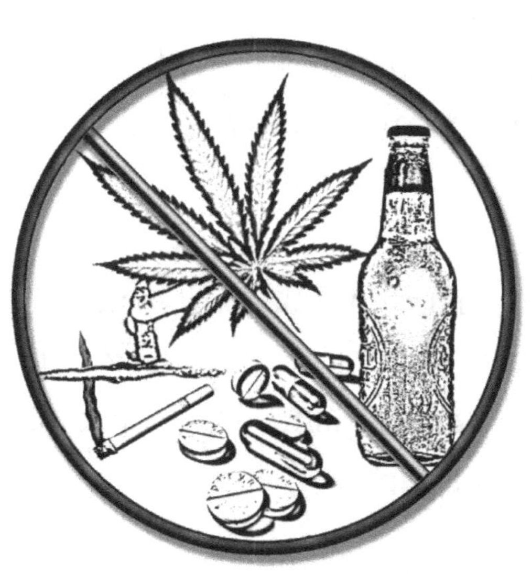

Purchasing or ordering Information: Amazon, Barnes & Noble, Ingram Spark, Apple, and your local bookstore.

For wholesale orders by U.S. trade bookstores chains and book distributors: please contact: dreammagicproductions@gmail.com

Printed in the United States of America

First Edition

14 13 12 11 10 / 10 9 8 7 6 5 4 3 2 1

Addiction: The Bible available in softcover from Amazon. It is available as an eBook from Smashwords.com

Introduction

The author/editor is a recovering alcoholic who has been in recovery for over 30 years. Early on his life, most of his friends and people who knew him believed that he was a hopeless case.

Early on, he felt this way also as his father had died of alcoholism and one f his half- brothers also died from his addictions.

I hope to be an example of recovery for everyone and anyone suffering from addiction.

No matter how bad things are and how seemingly hopeless your situation is, there is hope! There is always hope.

As the famous college coach, coach "V" is quoted as saying when he had terminal cancer: **"Never Give Up"**.

The following is a reprint of a powerful and in-depth article from the Huffington post. The Surgeon General's report follows this article followed by the alarming statistics on annual deaths by addiction in the US.

STAY WITH ME!

———

Huffington Post Reprint

CAUSE OF DEATH: ADDICTION?
MARCH 06, 2012
By Jeffrey B. Lane

The tragedy of Whitney Houston's early passing ignited the public's appetite for salacious television and print stories depicting celebrities "out of control." Unfortunately, this thirst for the sensational displays a profound misunderstanding of the disease of addiction and adds to the stigma attached to the disease already hidden behind a curtain of silence and a wealth of misunderstanding.

For all of the celebrities -- think Elvis Presley, Amy Winehouse, Heath Ledger, Jimi Hendrix, Janice Joplin, -- who suffered from addiction and were immortalized after death, there are over 100,000 ordinary Americans who die each year from the same disease and who will never become icons grieved by millions worldwide.

Yet their deaths bring the same shock and despair to their families and communities.

Today, over 80% of adult Americans suffer from one or more addictions.

Individuals can be addicted to: alcohol, nicotine, prescription or illicit drugs, and today, even FOOD!

Addiction is the largest preventable, most costly public health problem we face as a nation.

Approximately 50 % of our health care spending is driven by one of the above forms of addiction.

Across all government spending, the total financial cost is nearly $500 billion annually. And the human misery is incalculable.

It is long past time for public understanding of the disease of addiction to catch up with the science of this illness. Here's just a bit of what we now know:

Advances in neuroscience clearly demonstrate that addiction is a complex brain disease with significant behavioral characteristics. If untreated, it can become a chronic and relapsing condition that all too frequently ends in tragedy.

All addictive substances -- tobacco, alcohol, marijuana, opioids, stimulants, central nervous system depressants -- affect our brains.

More than 90 % of Americans who meet the medical criteria for addiction started smoking, drinking or using other drugs before age 18

. Because the teen brain is still developing, addictive substances physically alter its structure and function faster and more intensely than in adults, interfering with brain development, further impairing judgment and heightening the risk of addiction.

Certain individuals have personal characteristics or life circumstances that place them at even greater risk, including those with a genetic predisposition or a family history of addiction, those who have experienced abuse, neglect or other forms of trauma, and those with other mental health or behavioral conditions.

Culture, broadly defined, can increase the risk that individuals will use addictive substances. A wide range of social influences subtly condone or more overtly encourage use, including acceptance of substance misuse by peers, parents and communities; pervasive advertising of legally available products; media portrayals of substance use as benign or glamorous, fun and relaxing; and easy access to addictive substances.

Even with all this knowledge, addiction can be prevented, treated and managed effectively. But, as with other diseases, no one approach will work for all. New research results are enabling medical providers to tailor both pharmaceutical and behavior treatments according to the age, gender, disease severity, co-occurring conditions and the social and cultural circumstances of the affected individual. As with treatment for other diseases, this tailoring is critical to treatment success.

Although our scientific understanding of addiction has evolved, public attitudes and health care practice have not kept pace with this understanding.

The time has come to stop regarding addiction as a character flaw -- a personal and moral failing -- and to provide the treatment people suffering from the disease deserve, including long-term management for those with the chronic form of the disease, just as we do for hypertension or diabetes or cancer.

Why would we not do so? Imagine saying to a cancer patient: "We'll give you one course of treatment and if your cancer is not gone forever it's your fault." How many more of us must die before we strip the shame from the disease of addiction and properly respond to it as a debilitating and life-threatening medical problem?

Table of Contents

Chapter One

PREFACE FROM THE SURGEON GENERAL U.S. DEPARTMENT OF HEALTH AND HUMAN SERVICES

Before I assumed my position as U.S. Surgeon General, I stopped by the hospital where I had worked since my residency training to say goodbye to my colleagues. I wanted to thank them, especially the nurses, whose kindness and guidance had helped me on countless occasions. The nurses had one parting request for me. If you can only do one thing as Surgeon General, they said, please do something about the addiction crisis in America.

I have not forgotten their words. As I have traveled across our extraordinary nation, meeting people struggling with substance use disorders and their families, I have come to appreciate even more deeply something I recognized through my own experience in patient care: that substance use disorders represent one of the most pressing public health crises of our time.

Whether it is the rapid rise of prescription opioid addiction or the longstanding challenge of alcohol dependence, substance misuse and substance use disorders can—and do—prevent people from living healthy and productive lives. And, just as importantly, they have profound effects on families, friends, and entire communities.

I recognize that there is no single solution. We need more policies and programs that increase access to proven treatment modalities. We need to invest more in expanding the scientific evidence base for prevention, treatment, and recovery. We also need a cultural shift in how we think about addiction. For far too long, too many in our country have viewed addiction as a moral failing. This unfortunate stigma has created an added burden of shame that has made people with substance use disorders less likely to come forward and seek help. It has also made it more challenging to marshal the necessary investments in prevention and treatment. We must help everyone see that addiction is not a character flaw – it is a chronic illness that we must approach with the same skill and compassion with which we approach heart disease, diabetes, and cancer.

I am proud to release The Surgeon General's Report on Alcohol, Drugs, and Health. As the first ever Surgeon General's Report on this important topic, this Report aims to shift the way our society thinks about substance misuse and substance use disorders while defining actions we can take to prevent and treat these conditions.

Over the past few decades, we have built a robust evidence base on this subject. We now know that there is a neurobiological basis for substance use disorders with potential for both recovery and recurrence. We have evidence-based interventions that prevent harmful substance use and related problems, particularly when started early. We also have proven interventions for treating substance use disorders, often involving a combination of medication, counseling, and social support. Additionally, we have learned that recovery has many pathways that should be tailored to fit the unique cultural values and psychological and behavioral health needs of each individual.

As Surgeon General, I care deeply about the health and well-being of all who are affected by substance misuse and substance use disorders. This Report offers a way forward through a public health approach that is firmly grounded in the best available science. Recognizing that we all have a role to play, the Report contains suggested actions that are intended for parents, families, educators, health care professionals, public policy makers, researchers, and all community members.

Above all, we can never forget that the faces of substance use disorders are real people. They are a beloved family member, a friend, a colleague, and ourselves. Despite the significant work that remains ahead of us, there are reasons to be hopeful. I find hope in the people I have met in recovery all across America who are now helping others with substance use disorders find their way. I draw strength from the communities I have visited that are coming together to work on prevention initiatives and to connect more people to treatment. And I am inspired by the countless family members who have lost loved ones to addiction and who have transformed their pain into a passion for helping others. These individuals and communities are rays of hope. It is now our collective duty to bring such light to all corners of our country.

How we respond to this crisis is a moral test for America. Are we a nation willing to take on an epidemic that is causing great human suffering and economic loss? Are we able to live up to that most fundamental obligation we have as human beings: to care for one another?

Fifty years ago, the landmark Surgeon General's report on the dangers of smoking began a half century of work to end the tobacco epidemic and saved millions of lives. With the Surgeon General's Report on Alcohol, Drugs, and Health, I am issuing a new call to action to end the public health crisis of addiction. Please join me in taking the actions outlined in this Report and in helping ensure that all Americans can lead healthy and fulfilling lives.

Vivek H. Murthy, M.D., M.B.A.
Vice Admiral, U.S. Public Health Service
Surgeon General

EXECUTIVE SUMMARY

In 2015, over 27 million people in the United States reported current use of illicit drugs or misuse of prescription drugs, and over 66 million people (nearly a quarter of the adult and adolescent population) reported binge drinking in the past month. Alcohol and drug misuse and related disorders are major public health challenges that are taking an enormous toll on individuals, families, and society. Neighborhoods and communities as a whole are also suffering as a result of alcohol- and drug-related crime and violence, abuse and neglect of children, and the increased costs of health care associated with substance misuse. It is estimated that the yearly economic impact of substance misuse and substance use disorders is $249 billion for alcohol misuse and alcohol use disorders and $193 billion for illicit drug use and drug use disorders.

Despite the social and economic costs, this is a time of great opportunity. Ongoing health care and criminal justice reform efforts, as well as advances in clinical, research, and information technologies are creating new opportunities for increased access to effective prevention and treatment services. This Report reflects our commitment to leverage these opportunities to drive improvements in individual and public health related to substance misuse, use disorders, and related health consequences.

Binge drinking for men is drinking 5 or more standard alcoholic drinks, and for women, 4 or more standard alcoholic drinks on the same occasion on at least 1 day in the past 30 days.

The Many Consequences of Alcohol and Drug Misuse Alcohol and drug misuse can have a wide range of effects; a single instance of alcohol or drug misuse can have profound negative consequences. The specific effects associated with substance misuse depend on the substances used, how much and how often they are used, how they are taken (e.g., orally vs. injected), and other factors. Some of these effects include: Immediate, direct consequences: Substance misuse can have immediate, direct consequences for health ranging from effects on heart rate and regulation of body temperature to psychotic episodes, overdose, and death. Many more people now die from alcohol and drug overdoses each year than are killed in automobile accidents. The opioid crisis is fueling this trend with nearly 30,000 people dying due to an overdose on heroin or prescription opioids in 2014. An additional roughly 20,000 people died as a result of an unintentional overdose of alcohol, cocaine, or non-opioid prescription drugs.

Indirect consequences related to risky behaviors that often accompany alcohol and drug misuse: Alcohol and drug misuse can impair judgment, leading to risky behaviors including driving under the influence (DUI), unprotected sex, and needle/syringe sharing. Driving under the influence of alcohol or drugs contributes to thousands of deaths annually, and 10.6 percent of driver's report engaging in this hazardous behavior each year.

As misuse of some drugs such as prescription opioids progresses, many people seek to intensify the high by injecting them, and sharing of needles among users can result in outbreaks of HIV and hepatitis.

Longer-term health effects on a person's physical and mental health: For example, heavy drinking can lead to hypertension, liver disease, and cancer; regular marijuana use is associated with chronic bronchitis; and use of stimulants such as cocaine can lead to heart disease.

In addition, substance misuse during pregnancy can result in long lasting health effects for the baby including fetal alcohol spectrum disorders (FASDs), which are estimated to affect as many as 2 to 5 percent of the population, and neonatal abstinence syndrome (NAS); the ongoing opioid crisis has resulted in a five-fold increase in the number of babies who are dependent on opioids at birth.

Longer-term societal consequences: These can include reduced productivity, higher health care costs, unintended pregnancies, spread of infectious disease, drug-related crime, interpersonal violence, stress within families, and many other direct and indirect effects on communities, the economy, and society as a whole. Some of these consequences result from substance use disorders, which occur when a person uses alcohol or drugs to such an extent that it causes clinically significant impairments in health, social functioning, and voluntary control over substance use.

The majority of individuals who misuse substances do not develop a substance use disorder. However, roughly one in seven people in the United States (14.6 percent of the population) are expected to develop a substance use disorder at some point in their lives.

A substance use disorder can be diagnosed as mild, moderate, or severe depending on the extent of a person's symptoms. In this Report, addiction is used to refer to substance use disorders that can be categorized as severe and are associated with compulsive or uncontrolled use of one or more substances. Addiction is a chronic brain disease that, like milder substance use disorders, has the potential for both recurrence and recovery. In 2015, substance use disorders affected 20.8 million Americans—almost 8 percent of the adolescent and adult population. That number is similar to the number of people who suffer from diabetes, and more than 1.5 times the annual prevalence of all cancers combined (14 million). Of the 20.8 million people with a substance use disorder in 2015, 15.7 million were in need of treatment for an alcohol problem in 2015 and nearly 7.7 million needed treatment for an illicit drug problem.

Defined by the Centers for Disease Control and Prevention (CDC) as consuming 8 or more drinks per week for women, and 15 or more drinks per week for men, and by the Substance Abuse and

Mental Health Services Administration (SAMHSA), for research purposes, as binge drinking on 5 or more days in the past 30 days.

This Report follows the Fifth Edition of the Diagnostic and Statistical Manual of Mental Disorders, which defines substance use disorders as "clinically and functionally significant impairments caused by substance use, including health problems, disability, and failure to meet major responsibilities at work, school, or home."

Most Americans know someone with a substance use disorder, and many know someone who has lost or nearly lost a family member as a consequence of substance misuse. Yet, at the same time, few other medical conditions are surrounded by as much shame and misunderstanding as substance use disorders. Historically, our society has treated addiction and misuse of alcohol and drugs as symptoms of moral weakness or as a willful rejection of societal norms, and these problems have been addressed primarily through the criminal justice system. Our health care system has not given the same level of attention to substance use disorders as it has to other health concerns that affect similar numbers of people. Substance use disorder treatment in the United States remains largely segregated from the rest of health care and serves only a fraction of those in need of treatment. Only about 10 percent of people with a substance use disorder receive any type of specialty treatment. Further, over 40 percent of people with a substance use disorder also have a mental health condition, yet fewer than half (48.0 percent) receive treatment for either disorder.

Many factors contribute to this "treatment gap," including the inability to access or afford care, fear of shame and discrimination, and lack of screening for substance misuse and substance use disorders in general health care settings. Further, about 40 percent of individuals who know they have an alcohol or drug problem are not ready to stop using, and many others simply feel they do not have a problem or a need for treatment1— which may partly be a consequence of the neurobiological changes that profoundly affect the judgment, motivation, and priorities of a person with a substance use disorder.

Reasons for Hope and Optimism

The problem of alcohol and drug misuse in the United States is serious and pervasive. However, despite the challenges described above, this is also a time of great hope and opportunity:

$ Research on alcohol and drug use, and addiction, has led to an increase of knowledge and to one clear conclusion: Addiction to alcohol or drugs is a chronic but treatable brain disease that requires medical intervention, not moral judgment.

$ Policies and programs have been developed that are effective in preventing alcohol and drug misuse and reducing its negative effects.

$ Effective treatments for substance use disorders are available. Evidence-based treatments— both medications and behavioral therapies—can save lives and restore people's health, wellbeing, and functioning, as well as reduce the spread of infectious disease and lessen other consequences.

$ Support services such as mutual aid groups (e.g., Alcoholics Anonymous), recovery housing, and recovery coaches are increasingly available to help people in the long and often difficult task of maintaining recovery after treatment.

$ Health care reform efforts are creating new opportunities to increase access to prevention and treatment services to improve public health. Health insurers that participate in the new Health Care Marketplace must now cover costs related to mental health and substance use disorder services, including behavioral health treatment, and may not apply limitations on those benefits that are more restrictive than limitations applied on the benefits for medical and surgical services. Other incentives are encouraging general health systems to control costs, improve outcomes, and reduce readmissions by addressing patients' substance use. Transformations in the health care landscape are supporting integration of substance use disorder treatment with general health care in ways that will better address the needs of the millions of people suffering from these disorders.

$ The criminal justice system is engaged in efforts to place non-violent drug offenders in treatment instead of jail, to improve the delivery of evidence-based treatment for incarcerated persons, and to coordinate care in the community when inmates are released.

Together, these changes are leading to a new landscape of care for alcohol and drug misuse problems in America, and to new hope for millions of people who suffer from them.

Chapter Two

About Addiction

Addictive Substances and Addictive Behaviors

This chapter will provide an overview or a macro-cosmic perspective of the magnitude of the addiction crisis and the different addictive substances and behaviors that constitute the majority of the problem. Further chapters will examine the financial extend of the problem and the morbidity and mortality of this challenging situation.

•	Over 1 million people will needlessly die as a direct or indirect result of addiction in the US.

•	Addiction is a $1 trillion-dollar burden on the health care sectors (Government and private sectors).

•	Addiction in America is a cataclysmic problem and it looms as a colossal threat to the US economy and health care system.

•	Addiction has the potential to be the biggest health care catastrophe that the US has ever experienced. It is a problem that is growing exponentially.

•	Addiction is the leading cause of preventable death in the US.

•	The majority of the population of the United States will suffer from one or more addictions that often lead to death. Addiction negatively impacts every home and workplace.

The following page is a abbreviated list of the most common   addictive substances and addictive behaviors in the US.

Addictive Substances*

*Substance definition - A psychoactive compound with the potential to cause health and social problems, including substance use disorders (and their most severe manifestation, addiction).

Alcohol
Cannabis
Cocaine
Food
GHB (gamma-hydroxybutyric acid)
Heroin
Inhalants

Ketamine

LSD (lysergic acid diethylamide)

Marijuana (Cannabis)

MDMA (Ecstasy)

Mescaline (Peyote)

Methamphetamine

Nicotene (Cigarettes etc.)

Opioids

Over-the-counter Cough/Cold Medicines (Dextromethorphan or DXM)

PCP (Phencyclidine)

Prescription Opioids

Prescription Sedatives (Tranquilizers, Depressants)

Prescription drugs (sedatives, hypnotics, or anxiolytics like sleeping pills and tranquilizers)

Prescription Stimulants

Psilocybin

Rohypnol® (Flunitrazepam)

Steroids (Anabolic)

List of Addictive Behaviors

NOTE: The Diagnostic and Statistical Manual of Mental Disorders is used by clinicians and psychiatrists to diagnose psychiatric illnesses. In 2013, the latest version known as the DSM-5 was released. The DSM is published by the American Psychiatric Association and covers all categories of mental health disorders for both adults and children .addictive Behaviors

The DSM-5 lists disorders where impulses cannot be resisted, which are types of addictive behavior. The following is a partial list of the recognized impulse control disorders.

Listing of Impulse Control Addictive Behaviors

Intermittent explosive disorder (compulsive aggressive and assaultive acts)

Kleptomania (compulsive stealing)

Pyromania (compulsive setting of fires)

Gambling

Food (over-eating) -

Sex

Pornography (attaining, viewing)

Using computers / the internet

Playing video games

Working

Exercising

Spiritual obsession (as opposed to religious devotion)

Pain (seeking)

Cutting

Shopping

Chapter Three

Addiction Definitions

Several popular and accepted definitions of addiction follow.

Addiction is defined as a chronic, relapsing disorder characterized by compulsive drug seeking, continued use despite harmful consequences, and long-lasting changes in the brain. It is considered both a complex brain disorder and a mental illness.

Short Definition of Addiction: From ASAM – American Society of Addictive Medicine

Addiction is a primary, chronic disease of brain reward, motivation, memory and related circuitry. Dysfunction in these circuits leads to characteristic biological, psychological, social and spiritual manifestations. This is reflected in an individual pathologically pursuing reward and/or relief by substance use and other behaviors.

Addiction is characterized by inability to consistently abstain, impairment in behavioral control, craving, diminished recognition of significant problems with one's behaviors and interpersonal relationships, and a dysfunctional emotional response. Like other chronic diseases, addiction often involves cycles of relapse and remission. Without treatment or engagement in recovery activities, addiction is progressive and can result in disability or premature death.

What is addiction?

By Adam Felman   Reviewed by Vara Saripalli, PsyD

Addiction is a primary, chronic disease of brain reward, motivation, memory and related circuitry. Dysfunction in these circuits leads to characteristic biological, psychological, social and spiritual manifestations. This is reflected in an individual pathologically pursuing reward and/or relief by substance use and other behaviors.

Addiction is characterized by inability to consistently abstain, impairment in behavioral control, craving, diminished recognition of significant problems with one's behaviors and interpersonal relationships, and a dysfunctional emotional response. Like other chronic diseases, addiction often involves cycles of relapse and remission. Without treatment or engagement in recovery activities, addiction is progressive and can result in disability or premature death. Addiction is a psychological and physical inability to stop consuming a chemical, drug, activity, or substance, even though it is causing psychological and physical harm.

The term addiction does not only refer to dependence on substances such as heroin or cocaine. A person who cannot stop taking a particular drug or chemical has a substance dependence.

Some addictions also involve an inability to stop partaking in activities, such as gambling, eating, or working. In these circumstances, a person has a behavioral addiction.

Addiction is a chronic disease that can also result from taking medications.

The overuse of prescribed opioid painkillers, for example, causes 115 deaths every day in the United States.

When a person experiences addiction, they cannot control how they use a substance or partake in an activity, and they become dependent on it to cope with daily life.

Every year, addiction to alcohol, tobacco, illicit drugs, and prescription opioids costs the U.S. economy upward of $740 billion in treatment costs, lost work, and the effects of crime.

Most people start using a drug or first engage in an activity voluntarily. However, addiction can take over and reduce self-control.

- Not everyone that misuses a substance has an addiction.
- Drug addiction and drug misuse are different.
- Misuse refers to the incorrect, excessive, or non-therapeutic use of body- and mind-altering substances.
- However, not everybody that misuses a substance has an addiction. Addiction is the long-term inability to moderate or cease intake.
- For example, a person who drinks alcohol heavily on a night out may experience both the euphoric and harmful effects of the substance.
- However, this does not qualify as an addiction until the person feels the need to consume this amount of

alcohol regularly, alone, or at times of day when the alcohol will likely impair regular activities, such as in the morning.

A person who has not yet developed an addiction may put off further use by the harmful side effects of substance abuse. For example, vomiting or waking up with a hangover after drinking too much alcohol may deter some people from drinking that amount anytime soon.

Someone with an addiction will continue to misuse the substance despite the harmful effects.

Symptoms:

The primary indications of addiction are:

- uncontrollably seeking drugs -

• uncontrollably engaging in harmful levels of habit-forming behavior -

• neglecting or losing interest in activities that do not involve the harmful substance or behavior -

• relationship difficulties, which often involve lashing out at people who identify the dependency -

• an inability to stop using a drug, though it may be causing health problems or personal problems, such as issues with employment or relationships -

• hiding substances or behaviors and otherwise exercising secrecy, for example, by refusing to explain injuries that occurred while under the influence -

• profound changes in appearance, including a noticeable abandonment of hygiene-

• increased risk-taking, both to access the substance or activity and while using it or engaging in it -

- withdrawal – or withdrawal symptoms -
- depression -
- Stopping the use of a drug can lead to anxiety –

When a person has an addiction, and they stop taking the substance or engaging in the behavior, they may experience certain symptoms.

These symptoms may include:

Anxiety -
Irritability -
tremors and shaking –
nausea -
vomiting -
fatigue -
a loss of appetite –

- If a person has regularly used alcohol or benzodiazepines, and they stop suddenly or without medical supervision, withdrawal can be fatal.

Chapter Four

BioPsychoSocial-Model

This chapter is included in this tome for an important reason. The "sick" brain philosophy is becoming less important in the addictions field. The term "Evidence based recovery" is used a lot in the addictions field today, as well as the Surgeon General's very timely report. What "Evidence Based Recovery" means in the most simplistic terms is that after 1000's and 1000's of observations, professionals arrive at statistical conclusions as to what works and what doesn't.

What does work is taking a look at and analyzing the entire person, not just their brain. Essentially, mind and body are inseparable.

There are many biological indicators for addiction including genetic predisposition. The biopsychosocial model views health and illness as the product of biological characteristics (genes), behavioral factors (lifestyle, stress, health beliefs), and social conditions (cultural influences, family relationships, social support).

The biopsychosocial model is a modern humanistic and holistic view of the human being in health sciences. Currently, many researchers think the biopsychosocial model should be expanded to include the spiritual dimension as well. However, "spiritual" is an open and fluid concept, and it can refer to many different things.

Here we will explore the spiritual dimension in all its meanings: the spirituality-and-health relationship; spiritual–religious coping; the spirituality of the physician affecting his/her practice; spiritual support for inpatients; spiritual complementary therapies; and spiritual anomalous phenomena.

In order to ascertain whether physicians would be willing to embrace them all in practice, each phrase from the Physician's Pledge on the Declaration of Geneva (World Medical Association) was "translated" to its spiritual equivalent. Medical practice involves a continuous process of revisions of applied concepts, but a true paradigm shift will occur only when the human spiritual dimension is fully understood and incorporated into health care. Then, one will be able to cut stereotypes and use the term "biopsychosocial–spiritual model" correctly. A sincere and profound application of this new view of the human being would bring remarkable transformations to the concepts of health, disease, treatments, and cure.

The Biopsychosocial Model and the Spiritual Dimension

The biopsychosocial model is a modern humanistic and holistic view of the human being. The model was brought to medicine by George L. Engel (1913–1999), a prominent scholar engaged in the psychosomatic movement. As Engel stated: "all three levels, biological, psychological, and social, must be taken into account in every health care task". His claim was that physicians must simultaneously attend to the biological, psychological, and social dimensions of illness, in order to better understand and respond to patients' suffering.

At the practical level, it is a way of understanding the patient's subjective experience as an essential contributor to accurate diagnosis, health outcomes, and humane care". In the last decades, the humanization of medicine and empowerment of patients have been constantly improved by including the patient's subjective experience, by expanding the disease causational framework to a more comprehensive model, by valuating the patient–clinician relationship, and by giving new roles to the patient in clinical decision-making.

Currently, many researchers think the biopsychosocial model should be expanded to include the spiritual dimension as well. One such researcher's study has shown the relevance of spiritual symptoms and their interactions for understanding health outcomes.

Genuinely holistic health care must address the totality of the patient's relational existence. This will contribute to a more comprehensive model of care and research that takes account of patients in their fullest wholeness. Arguably, the transcendent and sacred questionings of the spiritual dimension cannot be exhausted on the mental and social grounds, notwithstanding the interfaces between the concepts.

"Health is a state of complete physical, mental and social well-being, and not merely the absence of disease or infirmity." In this definition, adopted in 1948 by the World Health Organization (WHO) after its foundation, the spiritual dimension was absent. However, in 1999, the 52nd Assembly of this institution proposed some amendments to its Constitution. One of the proposed modifications was the insertion of spiritual well-being into the WHO concept of health.

The new text would become "Health is a dynamic state of complete physical, mental, spiritual and social well-being and not merely the absence of disease or infirmity". Even so, despite approval during the Assembly, the new version was posteriorly vetoed. Notwithstanding, in many occasions on the last decades, the WHO highlighted the importance of the spiritual dimension for clinical purposes.

Chapter Five

Deaths by Addiction Type

When over a million people a year die as a result of various addictions, it is time that the "disease concept" needs to be applied. Addiction is not and should not be considered a moral and ethical failure or weakness on the part of its victims.

Addiction is every bit as much an illness as cancer, or diabetes, or a heart attack.

It is time that America moves out of the dark ages and addresses this epidemic just as it would any other disease or illness!

The following is the sad but accurate breakdown of addiction victims.

Smoking – Nicotine Cigarette smoking is responsible for more than 480,000 deaths per year in the United States, including more than 41,000 deaths resulting from secondhand smoke exposure. This is about one in five deaths annually, or 1,300 deaths every day. On average, smokers die 10 years earlier than nonsmokers.

FOOD*

*Addiction to food – Leading to health risks and death.

According Institutes of Health, obesity and overweight together are the second leading cause of preventable death in the United States, close behind tobacco use. An estimated 300,000 deaths per year are due to the obesity epidemic.

The results of two extensive studies examining obesity-attributable deaths in the United States were published in 1999. Allison, Fontaine, and Manson et al., reporting in the Journal of the American Medical Society, used data from a number of prospective cohort studies, including the Alameda Community Health Study, the Framingham Heart Study, the Tecumseh Community Health Study, the American Cancer Society's Cancer Prevention Study I, the National Health and Nutrition Examination Survey I Epidemiologic Follow-up Study, and the Nurses' Health Study, to estimate the number of deaths attributable to obesity in the United States on an annual basis. Their initial analyses, which examined deaths occurring among persons aged 18 and older in 1991, were adjusted only for age, sex, and smoking status. The weight categories used were overweight (BMI of 25-29.9), obese (BMI of 30-35), and severely obese (BMI >35).

Using data on all eligible subjects from all six studies, Allison et al. estimated that 280,184 obesity-attributable deaths occurred in the U.S. annually. When risk ratios calculated for nonsmokers and never-smokers were applied to the entire population (assuming these ratios to produce the best estimate for all subjects, regardless of smoking status, i.e., that obesity would exert the same deleterious effects across all smoking categories), the mean estimate for deaths due to obesity was 324,940.

Additional analyses were performed controlling for prevalent chronic disease at baseline using data from the CPS1 and

NHS. After controlling for preexisting disease, the mean annual number of obesity-attributable deaths was estimated to be 374,239 **(330,324** based on CPS1 data and **418,154** based on NHS data).

Alcohol-Related Deaths:

An estimated 88,000 people (approximately 62,000 men and 26,000 women) die from alcohol-related causes annually, making alcohol the third leading preventable cause of death in the United States. The first is tobacco, and the second is food addiction (including poor diet and physical inactivity).

In 2014, alcohol-impaired driving fatalities accounted for 9,967 deaths (31 percent of overall driving fatalities).

Alcohol-related deaths for young adults rose 68% between 2007 and 2017, while suicide deaths increased 35%. Rates for "deaths of despair" from alcohol, drugs and suicide were higher among young adults than among Baby Boomers and senior citizens.

Drug Overdose Deaths

More than 70,200 Americans died from drug overdoses in 2017, including illicit drugs and prescription opioids—a 2-fold increase in a decade. Drug overdose deaths rose from 16,849 in 1999 to 70,237 in 2017, a 400% plus increase.

Drug Overdose Death Rates – from the National Institute on Drug Abuse (NIDA) https://www.drugabuse.gov/related-topics/trends-statistics/overdose-death-rates

The number of drug deaths among young adults has risen by 400% in the past two decades, according to the non-profit America's Health and Well Being Trust. These deaths were fueled in large part by the opioid crisis, USA Today reports.

Cocaine – Cocaine is a type of psychostimulant that was involved in nearly 1 in 5 overdose deaths during 2017. Almost 5 million Americans reported current cocaine use in 2016, which is almost 2 percent of the population.

Cocaine-involved overdose death rates in the United States decreased from 2006-2012 but began increasing again in 2012 In 2017, drug overdose deaths involving cocaine increased by more than 34 percent, with almost **14,000** Americans dying from an overdose involving cocaine. From 2016-2017, among racial/ethnic groups the largest relative rate and absolute rate changes for cocaine-involved overdoses were highest among non-Hispanic blacks. Non-Hispanic blacks also experienced the highest death rate for overdoses involving cocaine in 2017.

The largest rate increases in cocaine-involved overdose death rates were in the Midwest region from 2016-2017. Overall, the 2017 rate was highest in the Northeast region. The highest death rates were in Washington D.C. and Ohio.

Heroin

Heroin-Related Overdose Deaths - As heroin use has increased, so have heroin-related overdose deaths:

During 2017, over 15,000 people died from drug overdoses involving heroin in the United States, a rate of almost 5 deaths for every 100,000 Americans.

Heroin-related overdose deaths increased five-fold from 2010 to 2017.

Inhalants

Every year an untold number of individuals die as a result of intentionally inhaling common, legal, everyday home, school and office products. The National Inhalant Prevention Coalition (NIPC) reports approximately 100 to 125 inhalant deaths per year, based on contacts with families of victims and media accounts. However this does not provide an accurate picture of the full extent of this public health problem.

Inhalant abuse related fatalities are underreported because they may not be recognized as such or because of a perceived stigma. Doctors and medical staff are traditionally one of the professions most focused on their continuing medical education using Medscape, medical journals, and other resources available to them, but even with all of that research it can be difficult for them to accurately identify signs of inhalant use. Therefore, The National Inhalant Prevention Coalition (NIPC) is providing background information and guidelines to assist medical examiners, coroners, pathologists and toxicologists to better understand, to recognize, to document and to accurately report inhalant deaths.

Ketamine

Ketamine is mentioned in this chapter for an interesting reason. As it becomes increasingly difficult to get prescriptions for opiates, people will search for new pain killers or solutions for pain relief.

Ketamine when combine with Tramadol provides a very powerful, but dangerous pain reliever. Ketamine is readily available as it is used in horse surgery.

An addiction to ketamine is difficult to overcome without help. Even when someone wants to stop using the drug, chemical changes in the brain make it nearly impossible to stop without professional help.

Once an individual crosses into the addicted state, they spend their days feeling utterly detached from their surroundings, and become incapable of leading a normal, productive life. They are usually cognitively impaired at this stage, with speech and memory both affected.

**Methamphetamine   -
Benzodiazepine overdose**

The federal government estimates that more than 10,000 people died of meth-related drug overdoses last year. Deaths from meth overdoses generally result from multiple organ failure or heart attacks and strokes, caused by extraordinary pulse rates and skyrocketing blood pressure.

In California, the number of amphetamine-related overdose deaths rose by 127 percent, from 456 in 2008 to 1,036 in 2013. At the same time, the number of opioid-related overdose deaths rose by 8.4 percent, from 1,784 to 1,934, according to the most recent data from the state Department of Public Health.

"It taxes your first responders, your emergency rooms, your coroners," according to a retired supervisor with the California Department of Justice. "It's an incredible burden on the health system."

Costs also are rising. A JAMA study, based on hospital discharge data, found that the cost of amphetamine-related hospitalizations had jumped from $436 million in 2003 to nearly $2.2 billion by 2015. Medicaid was the primary payer.

Benzodiazepines were involved in 31% of the estimated 22,767 deaths from prescription drug overdose in the United States. The US Food and Drug Administration (FDA) has subsequently issued a black box warning regarding concurrent use of benzodiazepines and opioids. Benzodiazepines are one of the most highly prescribed classes of drugs, and they are commonly used in self-poisoning.

Opioids

Opioid overdoses accounted for 42,000 deaths in 2016, more than any previous year. Over 40% of opioid deaths involved a prescription opioid!

Chapter Six

The "Why?" of Addiction

Why do some people become addicts and alcoholics?

- Genetics - It has been shown over and over that alcoholism and drug abuse runs in families.

Genes provide information on how our bodies respond at a cellular level. 99 percent of our genes are the same, while the 1 percent that are different account for things like hair and eye color, height, and even the potential for heart disease, diabetes or addiction to drugs and alcohol.

There is also evidence that the presence of specific genes, involved in alcohol metabolism and the transmission of nerve cell signals, increases the risk of becoming dependent on drugs or alcohol.

- Social Environment -

Social interactions and environmental circumstances fire up the brain's reward pathways.

As with most things, this can have both positive and negative effects on different individuals.

In cases where people live or attend school, or work in environments where alcohol and drugs are widely used to bond, it's been shown they're more likely to fall into patterns of substance abuse and addiction.

- Age of First Use -

Children who begin using alcohol or drugs before the age of 13 are 38% more likely to develop the disease of addiction.

Even moderate levels of abuse can damage their brains, which are generally not fully matured until the age of 25.

- Mental Illness -Half of drug abusers and about a third of alcoholics are also coping with a mental illness, such as depression or anxiety.

Likewise, half of those living with a severe mental illness, like bipolar disorder or schizophrenia, have substance abuse issues.

The existence of both mental illness and addiction is very common and referred to as dual diagnosis or co-occurring disorders.

- Early Childhood Trauma - Neglect, physical and emotional abandonment, sexual, physical and psychological abuse are all examples of trauma.

Scientists know that this kind of distress actually alters the brain chemistry of children and makes them more vulnerable to addiction later in life.

- Adult Trauma -This is similar to childhood trauma though it occurs later in life.

Those who suffer the loss of a loved one, such as a child, friend or spouse, or develop post-traumatic stress disorder (PTSD) as a result of combat experience, a car wreck or sexual assault have a propensity to self-medicate using drugs and alcohol.

This often leads to dependency and addiction.

Why do some people become addicted, while others do not?

No single factor can predict whether or not a person will become addicted to drugs. Risk for addiction is influenced by a person's biology, social environment, and age or stage of development. The more risk factors an individual has, the greater the chance that taking drugs can lead to addiction. According to the National Institute on Drug Abuse, the following three risk factors are most important:

- Biology - The genes that people are born with—in combination with environmental influences—account for about half of their addiction vulnerability. Additionally, gender, ethnicity, and the presence of other mental disorders may influence risk for drug abuse and addiction.

- Environment - A person's environment includes many different influences—from family and friends to socioeconomic status and quality of life in general. Factors such as peer pressure, physical and sexual abuse, stress, and parental involvement can greatly influence the course of drug abuse and addiction in a person's life.

- Development - Genetic and environmental factors interact with critical developmental stages in a person's life to affect addiction vulnerability, and adolescents experience a double challenge. Although taking drugs at any age can lead to addiction, the earlier that drug use begins, the more likely it is to progress to more serious abuse. And because adolescents' brains are still developing in the areas that govern decision making, judgment, and self-control, they are especially prone to risk-taking behaviors, including trying drugs of abuse.

Chapter Seven

What works?

Naltrexone? Acamprosate? AA? CBT?

Naltrexone -What is naltrexone?

Naltrexone is a medication that blocks the effects of drugs known as opiates, or narcotics (a class that includes morphine, heroin, or codeine). It competes with these drugs for opioid receptors in the brain. Originally used to treat dependence on opiate drugs, it now has also been approved by the U.S. Food and Drug Administration (FDA) as treatment for alcohol dependence. People who are dependent on opiate drugs, such as heroin or morphine, must stop their drug use at least 7 days prior to starting naltrexone. Some people should not take naltrexone, such as those suffering from chronic pain who rely on opioid painkillers or people with liver failure or acute hepatitis.

Although the precise mechanism of action for naltrexone's effect is unknown, reports from successfully treated patients suggest the following three kinds of effects:

- Naltrexone can reduce a patient's urge or desire to drink.
- Naltrexone helps patients remain abstinent.
- Naltrexone can interfere with the patient's desire to continue drinking more if he/she slips and has a drink.

In most clinical trials evaluating the effectiveness of naltrexone, subjects who received naltrexone were significantly more successful in remaining abstinent and in avoiding relapse than were those receiving an inactive placebo pill.

- Is it possible to become addicted to naltrexone?

No. Naltrexone is not habit forming or a drug of abuse. It does not cause users to become physically or psychologically dependent.

- What are the side effects of naltrexone?

In a large open-label safety study on naltrexone, conducted by Dupont Pharma in 570 individuals with alcoholism, the most common side effects affected only a small minority of people; they included the following:

Nausea (10 percent of participants)

Headache (7 percent of participants)

Depression (5 to 7 percent of participants)

Dizziness (4 percent of participants)

Fatigue (4 percent of participants)

Insomnia (3 percent of participants)

Anxiety (2 percent of participants

Sleepiness (2 percent of participants).

These side effects were usually mild and of short duration. Patients usually report that they are largely unaware of being on naltrexone. Naltrexone usually has no psychological effects, and users do not feel either "high" or "down." Naltrexone can have toxic effects on the liver. A patient receives blood tests of liver function prior to the onset of treatment and regularly during treatment to determine if he/she should take it at all, if he/she should stop taking it, or if he/she experiences the relatively rare side effect of liver toxicity. Patients should report any side effects to their medical clinician.

- What will happen if a patient drinks alcohol while taking naltrexone?

Naltrexone does not reduce the effects of alcohol that impair coordination and judgment. Naltrexone may reduce the feeling of intoxication and the desire to drink more, but it will not cause a severe physical response to drinking.

- Is it all right to take other medications with naltrexone?

Patients should carry a card explaining that they are taking naltrexone, and it should instruct medical staff on pain management. Naltrexone does not reduce the effectiveness of local and general anesthesia used with surgery. However, it does block pain relief from opiate medications. Many pain medications that are not opiates are available. Patients having elective surgery should stop taking naltrexone at least 72 hours beforehand.

The major active effect of naltrexone is on opiate (narcotic) drugs, which is one class of drugs used primarily to treat pain but is also found in some prescription cough preparations. Naltrexone will block the effect of normal doses of this type of drug. There are many nonnarcotic pain relievers patients can use while on naltrexone.

Otherwise, naltrexone is likely to have little impact on other medications patients commonly use such as antibiotics, nonopioid painkillers (e.g., aspirin, acetaminophen/Tylenol, buprofen/Motrin/Advil), and allergy medications. Patients should inform their medical clinician of the medication they are currently taking so that possible interactions can be evaluated. Because the liver breaks down naltrexone, other medications that can affect liver function may affect the dose of naltrexone.

- What will happen if a patient becomes pregnant while taking naltrexone?

Patients with the biological potential to have a child should be using an effective method of birth control while taking naltrexone. However, if they miss a menstrual period, they should report this to their medical clinician at once and take a pregnancy test.

If a patient becomes pregnant, she will discontinue the medication. The medical clinician should continue to ask after her health throughout her pregnancy as well as the health of her baby after delivery.

- Should naltrexone be taken with a meal?

There is no information that taking naltrexone with or without meals makes any difference in effect.

- What happens if a patient stops taking naltrexone suddenly?

Naltrexone does not cause physical dependence, and patients can stop taking it at any time without experiencing withdrawal symptoms.

- If patients take naltrexone, does it mean that they don't need other treatment for alcohol dependence?

No. Research studies have shown that naltrexone was most effective when it was combined with treatment from professionals and/or mutual-support groups.

- What is the relationship of naltrexone to AA and other support groups?

There is no contradiction between participating in support groups and taking naltrexone. In fact, one multisite study showed that naltrexone-taking subjects who attended mutual-support groups, such as AA, had better outcomes. It is most likely to be effective for patients whose goal is to stop drinking altogether. If other mutual-support group members caution against taking any medications, patients should refer them to the pamphlet "The AA Member—Medications and Other Drugs," which explicitly states that AA members should not "play doctor" and advise others on medication provided by legitimate, informed medical practitioners or treatment programs.

Acamprosate

What is acamprosate, and how does it work?

Acamprosate is a new, investigative medication for treatment of alcohol dependence approved in several European countries, and it is currently being studied in clinical trials in the United States. It is thought to reduce the urge for alcohol by working directly on certain neurotransmitters in the brain (chemicals that transmit information between nerve cells) whose balance has been disturbed because of regular, heavy drinking.

Although acamprosate can be used in the United States only with permission of the FDA, it has been available in Europe since 1989 and has recently been approved for marketing by prescription in more than 12 European countries, including Belgium, France, Germany, Ireland, Italy, the Netherlands, Spain, Switzerland, and the United Kingdom. It is estimated that more than 1 million patients have been treated with acamprosate since it became available.

Is acamprosate addictive?

No. Acamprosate is not habit forming or a drug of abuse. It does not cause users to become physically or psychologically dependent.

What are the side effects of acamprosate?

Like virtually all medications, acamprosate can cause side effects, but these are usually minor and go away as patients continue to take the medication. In European controlled clinical trials, the only types of symptoms that were consistently more common in subjects taking acamprosate than in subjects taking placebo were stomach symptoms. These were usually mild, tended to occur when subjects first started taking the medication, and consisted primarily of loose bowel movements or mild diarrhea. Some subjects also had changes in their sex drive—sometimes this was increased and sometimes decreased, but there was no definite pattern. As with many drugs, sometimes people on acamprosate develop skin rashes or itching. In earlier studies, subjects on acamprosate and those on placebo both experienced equal amounts of this type of symptom. Patients should tell their medical clinician of any side effects.

What will happen if a patient drinks alcohol while taking acamprosate?

Acamprosate does not change the way the body metabolizes alcohol, so acamprosate will not make patients feel sick if they drink (i.e., it does not work like Antabuse). In addition, there is no evidence of an added effect of alcohol if the patient drinks while taking acamprosate.

Is it okay to take other medications with acamprosate?

Because acamprosate is eliminated exclusively by the kidneys, drugs that may be toxic to the kidneys, such as aminoglycoside antibiotics (gentamycin and amikacin), should be avoided. Patients should inform their medical clinician of whatever medication they are currently taking so that possible interactions can be evaluated.

What will happen if a patient becomes pregnant while taking acamprosate?

Patients with the biological potential to have a child should be using an effective method of birth control while taking acamprosate. However, if they miss a menstrual period, they should report this to their medical clinician at once and take a pregnancy test.

If a patient becomes pregnant, she will discontinue the medication. The medical clinician should continue to ask after her health throughout her pregnancy as well as the health of her baby after delivery.

Even though acamprosate should not be used during pregnancy, animal studies have not shown any ill effects on either the course of pregnancy or on the offspring, nor is there any evidence from animal studies that acamprosate causes birth defects.

Should acamprosate be taken with a meal?

Acamprosate can be taken with food, but food does decrease the amount of medication that the body absorbs. Gastrointestinal symptoms may decrease by taking the medication with food.

Is it all right to crush the pills?

Acamprosate pills should not be crushed because they have an enteric coating. Destroying this coating can lead to a worsening of gastrointestinal side effects.

What happens if a patient stops taking acamprosate suddenly?

Acamprosate does not cause physiological withdrawal symptoms when it is stopped.

What happens if patients miss a dose?

If patients miss a dose of acamprosate, they should not take it simultaneously with the next scheduled dose; there should be a minimum of 2 hours between doses. If this is not feasible, they should not take the skipped dose. Instead, they should wait until their next scheduled dose and take only that dose.

If patients take acamprosate, does it mean that they don't need other treatment for alcohol dependence?

No. Research has shown that acamprosate was most effective when it was combined with treatment from professionals and/or mutual-support groups.

What is the relationship of acamprosate to AA and other mutual-support groups?

There is no contradiction between participating in support groups and taking acamprosate. It is most likely to be effective for patients whose goal is to stop drinking altogether. If other mutual-support group members caution against taking any medications, patients should refer them to the pamphlet "The AA Member—Medications and Other Drugs," which explicitly states that AA members should not "play doctor" and advise others on medication provided by legitimate, informed medical practitioners or treatment programs.

Chapter Eight

Future Trends

Trends that are Transforming the Field

U.S. News & World Report

Technology's New Role in Addiction Recovery

Doctors and scientists are harnessing modern technology to treat addiction.

By Robert Parkinson, Contributor -Jan. 3, 2017, at 6:00 a.m.

Technology's New Role in Addiction Recovery

IN 2016, PEOPLE RELY more and more on technology to make their lives easier in a variety of ways. Video communication is available to anyone with a cell phone or computer, virtual reality is becoming increasingly common and there seems to be an app for almost every need, no matter how obscure.

While many of these modern conveniences may seem frivolous at times, they're also being utilized by doctors and researchers to make people healthier. In fact, a number of the same tools people use to play games or chat with friends are also being put to use to combat alcohol and drug addiction, revolutionizing the way the disease is treated.

For example, just as there are apps for dating and food delivery, there are a number available designed to assist the recovery process, often at little or no cost to the user. The Alcoholics Anonymous

"Big Book" is currently available in the iTunes store, while Sober Grid helps patients find immediate support based on their current location. Other apps help track alcohol consumption or provide motivational messages to users, and some even employ the video functions on phones and computers to connect patients and physicians instantly.

Squirrel Recovery is another app that's making a great impact on addiction treatment. Developed at Ohio State University, it gives former addicts the opportunity to create their own support groups entirely based in a digital world. Members can check in on each other's well-being, and if someone is feeling low or at risk, their peers can offer immediate assistance.

Thanks to apps like Squirrel Recovery, Sober Grid and others, an entire support system is available at the push of a button – and anyone can access recovery assistance no matter how far they live from the nearest rehabilitation program.

Technology is also being harnessed at hospitals and treatment centers through various modern remedies. For instance, neurofeedback therapy is a developing method of training a patient's brain to stay centered at times they would otherwise crave alcohol or drugs. Using electrodes, laptops and special software, a doctor can read a patient's brainwaves and make decisions based on what he or she sees.

When the patient responds positively to a set of images, doctors will reward him or her with more positive reinforcement. Over time, the patients' brains learn to crave these rewards instead of alcohol or drugs.

Although neurofeedback therapy is a bit controversial, it has been embraced by rehabilitation programs. Others use different forms of cognitive behavioral therapy, which is considered a best practice in treating addiction. By changing the patterns that feed a person's addictions, addicts will learn how to change their attitudes toward and behaviors around alcohol and drugs.

At Virginia Tech, researchers have spent years working on computer programs that help addicts learn how to beat their addiction, but that also teach the patient about addiction over time.

By taking care of relaying the basic information about the disease, the computer program gives drug counselors more time to focus on individual needs instead. As a result, technology isn't just advantageous for recovering addicts – it also makes their caregivers' work much easier, which in turn benefits their patients in other ways.

Scientists are currently developing a number of other potential therapies that may one day prove to be extremely beneficial in addiction treatment. Virtual reality technology has expanded significantly in the last few years, and researchers in South Korea are employing the technique as medical care. In one study, test subjects watched three scenarios on a 3D television screen, including one that presented the unpleasant side effects of drinking, and the results were optimistic.

Meanwhile, the MIT Technology Review has written about fighting alcoholism with gene therapy. Using a genetic mutation common in East Asian populations, which causes a number of negative side effects in response to alcohol, researchers were able to compel rats not to crave alcohol. They're hoping to replicate the study in humans one day.

Gene therapy is extreme, and it will be years before it and other futuristic treatments are possible – if ever at all. Still, these advances prove that doctors and scientists are doing their best to harness modern technology for the purpose of treating addiction, building off innovations that may have been created for entirely different reasons. Today's dating app or self-driving car or video game could lead to tomorrow's cure for addiction. Only time will tell.

Addiction treatment has changed dramatically over the decades, but one thing has remained constant—there are no easy answers, either for those struggling with substance use disorders or those attempting to help them. Still, science gives us much to hope for, and accumulated experience is teaching us better each day what works and what doesn't.

Here are four predictions for what's just over the horizon in addiction treatment:

1. We will broaden our definition of success.

By moving away from our current focus on continuous abstinence as the only or best measure of success, we can build upon and celebrate every reduction in drug or alcohol use. The treatment process is then a journey, not a one-time shot at sobriety that the addicted person either passes or fails. It recognizes that people often relapse during the recovery process and that improvement most commonly comes over the long term.

With this more inclusive mindset must come a commitment to providing addiction treatment that follows the individual with a substance use problem through each stage of their journey. That, in turn, translates to less time spent using or drinking and, by extension, better quality of life, a decreased risk of overdose, lower rates of criminal behavior, less risk of sexually transmitted infections, and increased employment—all of which help not only the person in recovery but all those in their orbit.

2. Vaccines will supplement current treatments.

Medical advances promise a brave new world of addiction treatment that includes vaccines that can block or dampen the high from drugs. Already, clinical trials of a cocaine vaccine have indicated promise for creating "immunity" to cocaine. A heroin vaccine shows potential as well.

There are concerns: the protection may last only a limited time in some cases and some fear coercive use of vaccines. Still, for those struggling to put substance use behind them, vaccines could be a powerful tool.

3. We will stop treating every addiction in the same way.

Drugs of abuse either directly or indirectly affect the reward circuitry of the brain, and for that reason, they have been lumped in the same category. As a result, one-size-fits-all treatment has become the norm. It's an overly simplistic view that ignores the vast differences in the properties of various substances and their effects on those who use them.

The reality is all substances (and the people who use them) are not the same, and treatment shouldn't be either. Heroin addiction and alcohol addiction, for example, have different risks and challenges and should be approached in different ways. Recognizing this, as well as the reasons behind the person's substance use, will make success more likely and can head off negative consequences.

4. Treatment of co-occurring disorders will be paramount.

It's not always clear which came first, but it's now well-understood that addiction tends to go hand in hand with other disorders, such as depression, anxiety and trauma. Treating one demands a commitment to treating the other; otherwise a negative outcome is all but certain. Studies have found, for example, that depression quadruples the risk of relapse in alcoholics in the first year of recovery, and an 11-year study of heroin addicts found that mood disorders adversely affected every outcome in both the short and long term.

To provide effective help to those with co-occurring disorders, the skills and training of substance abuse counselors must expand. In addition, it's crucial that fully integrated psychiatric and mental health diagnosis and treatment be provided at every level of addiction care. It's a future that won't come easy, but it's one that will be well worth the effort.

Appendix A – listing of addiction organizations

Important Federal, State, and Private Addiction Organizations

The following organization provide among other things invaluable - in-depth and state-of-the art understandings of addiction, addictive behavior, the history of addiction, as well as information critical to recovery and where to get help.

SAMSHA

Who is SAMSHA? What is SAMSHA?

The SAMSHA web site provides links and phone numbers to many helpful services. It can be an invaluable resource to both clinicians and for people that seek help and need access to important resources.

The Substance Abuse and Mental Health Services Administration (SAMHSA) is the agency within the U.S. Department of Health and Human Services that leads public health efforts to advance the behavioral health of the nation. SAMHSA's mission is to reduce the impact of substance abuse and mental illness on America's communities.

Seeking treatment options? Feel free to use the SAMSHA help phone line.

Help is available in both English and Spanish. Learn more about the SAMHSA National Helpline.

1-800-662-HELP (4357)

TTY: 1-800-487-4889

SAMHSA New Social Media Accounts

Facebook

SAMHSA's Facebook page seeks to reduce the impact of substance abuse and mental illness on America's communities. Facebook comments and likes allow people to interact with SAMHSA concerning public health topics.

SAMSHA on Twitter

HHS on Twitter

SAMHSA tweets about news, webinars, videos, hotlines, grants, special programs, and activities. The hashtag directory tells you which hashtags SAMHSA uses to target specific topics and audiences. Please join SAMHSA's conversations!

The Blog SAMHSA Blog

The SAMHSA blog is written by SAMHSA staff. Blog articles give clear, up-to-date explanations of behavioral health topics, new programs, recent reports, and current grant opportunities. Dialogue is the perfect place to discover the latest resources and share ideas with others in the health care world.

NIH – National Institute of Health

The NIH is more than likely the largest and most influential organization when it comes to addiction.

The following information is quite revealing as to the understanding of drug, alcohol and behavior addiction in the US.

U.S. Department of Health & Human Services

National Institutes of Health (NIH)

We were only beginning to understand how drugs of abuse worked in the brain, as the technologies that would reveal how and which brain areas were affected in humans were just coming into use.

The wide-ranging health effects of drug abuse (e.g., heart and lung diseases, hepatitis and HIV/AIDS) were also just being discovered.

Methadone was the only medication available for treating drug addiction. Behavioral treatments existed but were not yet in use.

Brain imaging technology has demonstrated that addiction is a brain disease by delineating profound disruptions in the specific brain circuits affected by addiction. These changes go beyond the brain's reward system to include regions involved in memory, learning, impulse control, stress reactivity, and more. Repeated drug exposure "resets" these circuits toward compulsive behavior so that a person's control over the desire to seek and use drugs is compromised, despite devastating consequences.

NIAAA (Another subset or division of NIH)

About NIAAA

The National Institute on Alcohol Abuse and Alcoholism (NIAAA) is one of the 27 institutes and centers that comprise the National Institutes of Health (NIH). NIAAA supports and conducts research on the impact of alcohol use on human health and well-being. It is the largest funder of alcohol research in the world.

NIAAA leads the national effort to reduce alcohol-related problems by:

Conducting and supporting alcohol-related research in a wide range of scientific areas including genetics, neuroscience, epidemiology, prevention, and treatment.

Coordinating and collaborating with other research institutes and federal programs on alcohol-related issues.

Collaborating with international, national, state, and local institutions, organizations, agencies, and programs engaged in alcohol-related work.

Translating and disseminating research findings to health care providers, researchers, policymakers, and the public.

Through both research within NIAAA, and by funding grants at institutions worldwide, NIAAA aims to:

Better understand the health effects of alcohol consumption, including why it can cause addiction.

Reveal the biological and socio-cultural origins of why people respond to alcohol differently.

Remove the stigma associated with alcohol problems.

Develop effective prevention and treatment strategies that address the physical, behavioral, and social risks that result from both excessive alcohol use, and underage alcohol consumption.

Projects & Initiatives

NIAAA promotes advancement in several critical research areas with special programs and by participating on select committees. Priority research areas include:

Medications Development

NIAAA's Medications Development Program focuses on expanding safe and effective medication options for those suffering from alcohol use disorders and alcohol induced organ damage. The Medications Development Program offers funding grants and contracts to academic research institutions and small businesses developing novel medication treatments.

NIDA – National Institute on Drug Abuse

NIDA Ensuring the effective translation, implementation, and dissemination of scientific research findings to improve the prevention and treatment of substance use disorders and enhance public awareness of addiction as a brain disorder.

The Science of Addiction – NIDA publication

Preface:

How Science Has Revolutionized the Understanding of Drug Addiction

For much of the past century, scientists studying drugs and drug use labored in the shadows of powerful myths and misconceptions about the nature of addiction. When scientists began to study addictive behavior in the 1930s, people addicted to drugs were thought to be morally flawed and lacking in willpower. Those views shaped society's responses to drug use, treating it as a moral failing rather than a health problem, which led to an emphasis on punishment rather than prevention and treatment.

Drugs of Abuse–(NIDA perspective)
Cocaine
Heroin
Marijuana
MDMA (Ecstasy)
Methamphetamine
Opioids
Prescription Medicines

Treatment Information - NIDA does not provide medical advice. For medical advice, we strongly urge you to contact a qualified health care provider.

For information about how to know if you or a loved one needs treatment, and how to find it, visit our Step-by-Step Guides.

To find a treatment center in your area, please visit the SAMHSA Treatment Locator. NIDA does not endorse any specific treatment program.

If you are looking for an addiction specialist, please visit the American Society of Addiction Medicine.

Still Have Questions for Our Staff?

Complete our Contact NIDA form, and we will try to help. Please submit your query through only the Contact NIDA form; do not also send the same query through other email addresses found on the NIDA site. We will route your message to the appropriate contact and try to respond within 3 to 5 business days.

For Mail Inquiries Regarding NIDA

National Institute on Drug Abuse
Office of Science Policy and Communications

Public Information and Liaison Branch

6001 Executive Boulevard
Room 5213, MSC 9561
Bethesda, Maryland 20892

For Phone Inquiries

301-443-1124

Contact Us:

USA.gov   HHS   NIH
www.drugabuse.gov/

We lift the voices of those impacted by substance use to eliminate the stigma around addiction in our country. We're creating a movement to extinguish the deep-rooted misperceptions that surround addiction and prevent our society from investing the resources required to ensure no family loses a child to substance use or addiction.

WHO

(World Health Organization)

WHO International statistics on alcohol abuse and Alcohol abuse morbidity and alcohol abuse mortality.

Harmful use of alcohol kills more than 3 million people each year, most of them men

21 September 2018 News release

More than 3 million people died as a result of harmful use of alcohol in 2016, according a report released by the World Health Organization (WHO) today. This represents 1 in 20 deaths. More than three quarters of these deaths were among men. Overall, the harmful use of alcohol causes more than 5% of the global disease burden.

WHO's Global status report on alcohol and health 2018 presents a comprehensive picture of alcohol consumption and the disease burden attributable to alcohol worldwide. It also describes what countries are doing to reduce this burden.

"Far too many people, their families and communities suffer the consequences of the harmful use of alcohol through violence, injuries, mental health problems and diseases like cancer and stroke," said Dr Tedros Adhanom Ghebreyesus, Director-General of WHO. "It's time to step up action to prevent this serious threat to the development of healthy societies."

Of all deaths attributable to alcohol, 28% were due to injuries, such as those from traffic crashes, self-harm and interpersonal violence; 21% due to digestive disorders; 19% due to cardiovascular diseases, and the remainder due to infectious diseases, cancers, mental disorders and other health conditions.

Globally an estimated 237 million men and 46 million women suffer from alcohol-use disorders with the highest prevalence among men and women in the European region (14.8% and 3.5%) and the Region of Americas (11.5% and 5.1%). Alcohol-use disorders are more common in high-income countries.

Global consumption predicted to increase in the next 10 years

An estimated 2.3 billion people are current drinkers. Alcohol is consumed by more than half of the population in three WHO regions – the Americas, Europe and the Western Pacific.

Worldwide, more than a quarter (27%) of all 15–19-year-olds are current drinkers. Rates of current drinking are highest among 15–19-year-olds in Europe

(44%), followed by the Americas (38%) and the Western Pacific (38%). School surveys indicate that, in many countries, alcohol use starts before the age of 15 with very small differences between boys and girls.

Appendix B

Addiction terms and terminology

Glossary - Commonly Used Terms in Addiction Science

A

Abstinence: Not using drugs or alcohol.

Addiction: A chronic, relapsing disorder characterized by compulsive (or difficult to control) drug seeking and use despite harmful consequences, as well as long-lasting changes in the brain. In the past, people who used drugs were called "addicts." Current appropriate terms are people who use drugs and drug users.

Agonist: A chemical substance that binds to and activates certain receptors on cells, causing a biological response. Oxycodone, morphine, heroin, fentanyl, methadone, and endorphins are all examples of opioid receptor agonists.

Amphetamine: A stimulant drug that acts on the central nervous system (CNS). Amphetamines are medications prescribed to treat attention deficit hyperactivity disorder (such as Adderall®) and narcolepsy.

Anabolic-androgenic steroids: Synthetic substances similar to the male hormone testosterone. Often known as "anabolic steroids." They can promote muscle growth (anabolic effects) and produce changes in male sexual characteristics (androgenic effects) in both males and females.

Analgesics: A group of medications that reduce pain.

Anesthetic: A drug that causes insensitivity to pain and is used for surgeries and other medical procedures.

Antagonist: A chemical substance that binds to and blocks the activation of certain receptors on cells, preventing a biological response. Naloxone is an example of an opioid receptor antagonist.

B

Barbiturate: A type of CNS depressant sometimes prescribed to promote relaxation and sleep, but more commonly used in surgical procedures and to treat seizure disorders.

Basal ganglia: The area of the brain that plays an important role in positive forms of motivation, including the pleasurable effects of healthy activities like eating, socializing, and sex, and are also involved in the formation of habits and routines. These areas form a key node of what is sometimes called the brain's "reward circuit."

Benzodiazepine: A type of CNS depressant sometimes prescribed to relieve anxiety, panic, or acute stress reactions. Some benzodiazepines are prescribed short-term to promote sleep. Diazepam (Valium®) and alprazolam (Xanax®) are among the most widely prescribed benzodiazepine medications.

Brainstem: A group of brain structures that process sensory information and control basic functions needed for survival such as breathing, heart rate, blood pressure, and arousal.

Buprenorphine: An opioid partial agonist medication prescribed for the treatment of opioid addiction that relieves drug cravings without producing the high or dangerous side effects of other opioids.

C

Cannabidiol (CBD): A component of the marijuana plant without mind-altering effects that is being studied for possible medical uses.

Cannabinoid receptor: The receptor in the brain that recognizes and binds cannabinoids that are produced in the brain (anandamide) or outside the body (THC).

Cannabinoids: Chemicals that bind to cannabinoid receptors in the brain. They are found naturally in the brain (anandamide, 2-arachidonoylglycerol) and also in marijuana (THC and CBD). They are involved in a variety of mental and physical processes, including memory, thinking, concentration, movement, pain regulation, food intake, and reward.

Cannabis: Another name for the marijuana plant, Cannabis sativa.

Cardiovascular system: The system consisting of the heart and blood vessels. It delivers nutrients and oxygen to all cells in the body.

Central nervous system (CNS): The system consisting of the nerves in the brain and spinal cord.

Cerebellum: A part of the brain that helps regulate posture, balance, and coordination. It is also involved in the processes of emotion, motivation, memory, and thought.

Cerebral cortex: The gray matter that covers the surface of the cerebral hemispheres, whose functions include sensory processing and motor control along with language, reasoning, decision-making, and judgment.

Cerebral hemispheres: The right and left halves of the brain.

Cerebrum: The upper part of the brain consisting of the left and right hemispheres.

CNS depressants: A class of drugs that include sedatives, tranquilizers, and hypnotics. These drugs slow brain activity, making them useful for treating anxiety, panic, acute stress reactions, and sleep disorders.

Cognition (n): Of or relating to the act or process of thinking, understanding, learning, and remembering.

Cognitive-behavioral therapy (CBT): A form of psychotherapy that teaches people strategies to identify and correct problematic associations among thoughts, emotions, and behaviors in order to enhance self-control, stop drug use, and address a range of other problems that often co-occur with them.

Comorbidity: When two disorders or illnesses occur in the same person. Drug addiction and other mental illnesses or viral infections (HIV, hepatitis) are often comorbid. Also referred to as co-occurring disorders.

Contingency management: A treatment approach based on providing incentives to support positive behavior change.

Craving: A powerful, often overwhelming desire to use drugs.

D

Dependence: A condition that can occur with the regular use of illicit or some prescription drugs, even if taken as prescribed. Dependence is characterized by withdrawal symptoms when drug use is stopped. A person can be dependent on a substance without being addicted, but dependence sometimes leads to addiction.

Detoxification: A process in which the body rids itself of a drug, or its metabolites. Medically-assisted detoxification may be needed to help manage a person's withdrawal symptoms. Detoxification alone is not a treatment for substance use disorders, but this is often the first step in a drug treatment program.

Dopamine: A brain chemical, classified as a neurotransmitter, found in regions of the brain that regulate movement, emotion, motivation, and reinforcement of rewarding behavior. Dopamine release in reward areas of the brain is caused by all drugs to which people can become addicted.

Drug abuse: An older diagnostic term that defined use that is unsafe, use that leads a person to fail to fulfill responsibilities or gets them in legal trouble, or use that continues despite causing persistent interpersonal problems. This term is increasingly avoided by professionals because it can perpetuate stigma. Current appropriate terms include: drug use (in the case of illicit substances), drug misuse (in the case of problematic use of legal drugs or prescription medications) and addiction (in the case of substance use disorder).

Drugged driving: Driving a vehicle while impaired due to the intoxicating effects of recent drug use.

E

Electronic cigarette: A battery-operated device that people use to inhale an aerosol, which typically contains nicotine, flavorings, and other chemicals; also called e-cigarette, e-cigs, e-vaporizers, or electronic nicotine delivery system.

F

Flashback: A sudden but temporary recurrence of aspects of a drug experience (including sights, sounds, and feelings) that may occur days, weeks, or even more than a year after using drugs that cause hallucinations.

H

Hallucinations: Sensations, sounds and/or images that seem real though they are not.

Hippocampus: An area of the brain crucial for learning and memory.

Hypothalamus: A part of the brain that controls many bodily functions, including eating, drinking, body temperature regulation, and the release of many hormones.

I

Illicit: Illegal or forbidden by law.

Impulsivity: A tendency to act without foresight or regard for consequences and to prioritize immediate rewards over long-term goals.

Injection drug use (IDU): The act of administering drugs by injection. Blood-borne viruses, like HIV and hepatitis, can be transmitted via shared needles or other drug injection equipment.

Intranasal: Taken through the nose.

L

Limbic system: Interconnected brain structures that process feelings, emotions, and motivations. It is also important for learning and memory.

M

Mental disorder: A mental condition marked primarily by disorganization of personality, mind, and emotions that seriously impairs the psychological or behavioral functioning of the individual. This is sometimes referred to as a mental health condition. Addiction is a mental disorder.

Methadone: A long-acting opioid agonist medication used for the treatment of opioid addiction and pain. Methadone used for opioid addiction can only be dispensed by opioid treatment programs certified by SAMHSA and approved by the designated state authority.

Motivational Enhancement Therapy: A counseling approach that uses motivational interviewing techniques to help individuals resolve any uncertainties they have about stopping their substance use. The therapy helps the person strengthen their own plan for change and engagement in treatment.

N

Naloxone: An opioid antagonist medication approved by the FDA to reverse an opioid overdose. It displaces opioid drugs (such as morphine or heroin) from their receptor and prevents further opioid receptor activation.

Naltrexone: A long-acting opioid antagonist medication that prevents receptors from being activated by other opioids. Naltrexone is used to treat alcohol and opioid use disorders.

Neonatal Abstinence Syndrome (NAS): A condition of withdrawal that occurs when certain drugs pass from the mother through the placenta into the fetus' bloodstream during pregnancy causing the baby to become drug dependent and experience withdrawal after birth. The type and severity of a baby's withdrawal symptoms depend on the drug(s) used, how long and how often the mother used, how her body broke down the drug, and if the baby was born full term or prematurely. NAS can require hospitalization and treatment with medication to relieve symptoms.

Neurobiology: The study of the anatomy, function, and diseases of the brain and nervous system.

Neuron (nerve cell): A unique type of cell found in the brain and throughout the body that specializes in the transmission and processing of information.

Neurotransmitter: A chemical compound that acts as a messenger to carry signals from one nerve cell to another.

Norepinephrine: A neurotransmitter that affects heart rate, blood pressure, stress, and attention.

Nucleus accumbens: A brain region in the ventral striatum involved in motivation and reward. Nearly all addictive drugs directly or indirectly increase dopamine in the nucleus accumbens, contributing to their addictive properties.

O

Opioid receptors: Proteins on the surface of neurons, or other cells, that are activated by endogenous opioids, such as endorphins, and opioid drugs, such as heroin. Opioid receptor subtypes include mu, kappa, and delta.

Overdose: An overdose occurs when a person uses enough of a drug to produce a life-threatening reaction or death.

P

Paranoia: Extreme and unreasonable distrust of others.

Partial agonist: A substance that binds to and activates a receptor to a lesser degree than a full agonist.

Pharmacodynamics: The way a drug acts on the body. This includes the drug's interaction with its biological target and the resulting changes (such as activation or blocking of receptors), as well as the relationship between drug dosing and drug effects.

Pharmacokinetics: What the body does to a drug after it has been taken, including how rapidly the drug is absorbed, broken down, and processed by the body.

Pharmacotherapy: Treatment using medications.

Prefrontal cortex: The front part of the brain responsible for reasoning, planning, problem solving, and other higher cognitive functions. This area of the brain is not fully mature until adulthood, which confers greater vulnerability to drug use on the adolescent brain.

Prescription drug misuse: The use of a medication in ways or amounts other than intended by a doctor, by someone other than for whom the medication is prescribed, or for the experience or feeling the medication causes. This term is used interchangeably with "nonmedical" use, a term employed by many national drug use surveys.

Psychedelic drug: A drug that distorts perception, thought, and feeling. This term is typically used to refer to drugs with hallucinogenic effects.

Psychoactive: Having a specific effect on the brain.

Psychosis: Delusional or disordered thinking detached from reality; symptoms often include hallucinations.

Psychotherapeutics: Drugs that have an effect on the function of the brain and that are often used to treat psychiatric/neurologic disorders; includes pain relievers, tranquilizers, sedatives, and stimulants.

Psychotropic: Mind-altering.

R

Receptor: A molecule located on the surface of a cell that recognizes specific chemicals (normally neurotransmitters, hormones, and similar endogenous substances) and transmits the chemical message into the cell.

Recovery: A process of change through which people with substance use disorders improve their health and wellness, live self-directed lives, and strive to reach their full potential.

Relapse: In drug addiction, relapse is the return to drug use after an attempt to stop. Relapse is a common occurrence in many chronic health disorders, including addiction, that requires frequent behavioral and/or pharmacologic adjustments to be treated effectively.

Remission: A medical term meaning that major disease symptoms are eliminated or diminished below a pre-determined harmful level.

Reward: Pleasurable feelings that reinforce behavior and encourage repetition.

Reward system (or brain reward system): A brain circuit that includes the ventral tegmental area, the nucleus accumbens, and the prefrontal cortex.

Risk factors: Factors that increase the likelihood of beginning substance use, of regular and harmful use, and of other behavioral health problems associated with use.

Route of administration: The way a drug is taken into the body. Drugs are most commonly taken by eating, drinking, inhaling, injecting, snorting, or smoking.

Self-medication: The use of a substance to lessen the negative effects of stress, anxiety, or other mental disorders (or side effects of their pharmacotherapy) without the guidance of a health care provider. Self-medication may lead to addiction and other drug- or alcohol-related problems.

Serotonin: A neurotransmitter involved in a broad range of effects on perception, movement, and emotions. Serotonin and its receptors are the targets of most hallucinogens.

Stigma: A set of negative attitudes and beliefs that motivate people to fear and discriminate against other people. Many people do not understand that addiction is a disorder just like other chronic disorders. For these reasons, they frequently attach more stigma to it. Stigma, whether perceived or real, often fuels myths and misconceptions, and can influence choices. It can impact attitudes about seeking treatment, reactions from family and friends, behavioral health education and awareness, and the likelihood that someone will not seek or remain in treatment.

Substance use disorder (SUD): A medical illness caused by disordered use of a substance or substances. According to the Fifth Edition of the Diagnostic and Statistical Manual of Mental Disorders (DSM-5), SUDs are characterized by clinically significant impairments in health, social function, and impaired control over substance use and are diagnosed through assessing cognitive, behavioral, and psychological symptoms. An SUD can range from mild to severe.

T

THC: Delta-9-tetrahydrocannabinol; the main mind-altering ingredient in marijuana.

Tolerance: A condition in which higher doses of a drug are required to achieve the desired effect.

V

Vaping: Inhaling the aerosol or vapor from an electronic cigarette, e-vaporizer, or other device.

Ventral striatum: An area of the brain that is part of the basal ganglia and includes the nucleus accumbens; dopamine is released here in the presence of salient stimuli and in response to physically rewarding activities such as eating, sex, and taking drugs, and this process is a key factor behind the desire to repeat the behaviors associated with these rewarding activities.

Ventral tegmental area: An area in the brainstem that contains dopamine neurons that make up a key part of the brain reward system, which also includes the nucleus accumbens and prefrontal cortex.

W

Withdrawal: Symptoms that can occur after long-term use of a drug is reduced or stopped; these symptoms occur if tolerance to a substance has occurred, and vary according to substance. Withdrawal symptoms can include negative emotions such as stress, anxiety, or depression, as well as physical effects such as nausea, vomiting, muscle aches, and cramping, among others. Withdrawal symptoms often lead a person to use the substance again.

Notes: